中国结核病防治

生态图集

主审　刘剑君

主编　赵雁林

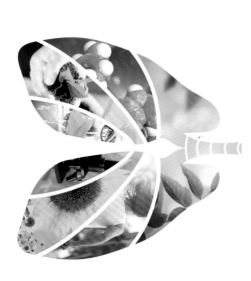

人民卫生出版社
·北京·

图书在版编目（CIP）数据

中国结核病防治生态图集 / 赵雁林主编. —北京：
人民卫生出版社，2021.10
ISBN 978-7-117-32138-9

Ⅰ．①中… Ⅱ．①赵… Ⅲ．①结核病 – 防治 – 图集
Ⅳ．①R52-64

中国版本图书馆 CIP 数据核字（2021）第 194820 号

| 人卫智网 | www.ipmph.com | 医学教育、学术、考试、健康， | 购书智慧智能综合服务平台 |
| 人卫官网 | www.pmph.com | 人卫官方资讯发布平台 |

中国结核病防治生态图集
Zhongguo Jiehebing Fangzhi Shengtaituji

主　　编：	赵雁林
出版发行：	人民卫生出版社（中继线 010-59780011）
地　　址：	北京市朝阳区潘家园南里 19 号
邮　　编：	100021
E - mail：	pmph @ pmph.com
购书热线：	010-59787592　010-59787584　010-65264830
印　　刷：	北京华联印刷有限公司
经　　销：	新华书店
开　　本：	787×1092　1/16　　印张：3.5
字　　数：	63 千字
版　　次：	2021 年 10 月第 1 版
印　　次：	2021 年 11 月第 1 次印刷
标准书号：	ISBN 978-7-117-32138-9
定　　价：	65.00 元

| 打击盗版举报电话：010-59787491 | E-mail：WQ @ pmph.com |
| 质量问题联系电话：010-59787234 | E-mail：zhiliang @ pmph.com |

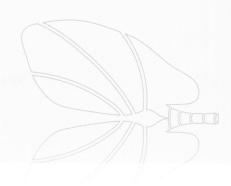

《中国结核病防治生态图集》编写委员会

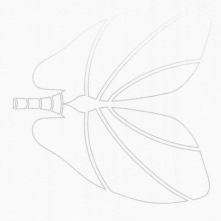

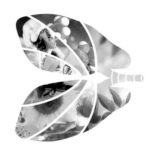

前 言

结核病是严重危害人民群众身心健康的重大传染病，是传染病中的头号杀手。我国结核病疾病负担位居全球第三位，每年新增报告肺结核患者约70万例，位居甲乙类传染病中的第二位，再加上人口老龄化、人口流动等因素，结核病防治形势依然十分严峻。

我国党和政府历来高度重视结核病防治工作，近年来陆续出台一系列政策、规范和技术指南。《"健康中国2030"规划纲要》和《健康中国行动(2019—2030年)》都明确提出重大传染病防控，强调要建立结核病防治综合服务模式，加强耐药肺结核筛查和监测，规范肺结核诊疗管理，保持全国肺结核疫情持续下降。为进一步贯彻落实《"健康中国2030"规划纲要》，国家卫生健康委等八部委联合下发了《遏制结核病行动计划(2019—2022年)》，2020年国家卫生健康委印发了《中国结核病预防控制工作技术规范(2020年版)》，并联合教育部制定了《中国学校结核病防控指南》。这一系列的规范和指南，是我国未来一段时间内结核病防治的纲领性文件。

为了便于大家更好地理解、准确地掌握并有效地落实上述各项规范、指南，中国疾病预防控制中心结核病预防控制中心广泛征求各级结核病防治专业机构(疾控机构)、医疗机构和基层医疗卫生机构、科研院所和学术团体等相关领域专家的建议和意见，组织编写了《中国结核病防治生态图集》(以下简称《生态图》)。《生态图》简明生动、全方位立体展示了目前我国结核病防治工作的主要环节，内容涉及结核病防治的全链条、全过程，涵盖了结核防治策略、技术措施、相关机构的主要任务和结核病防治工作各项具体措施及质量控制的关键流程。《生态图》不仅可以供各级卫生健康行政部门、疾病预防控制机构、医疗机构以及基层医疗卫生机构从事结核病防治工作的人员使用，也可以供卫生系统之外的相关人士参考。《生态图》同时提供了中文和英文两个版本，方便各级相关机构对外交流和国际友人分享中国经验。

编者

2021 年 8 月

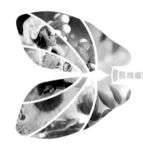

目 录

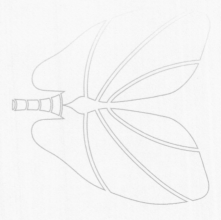

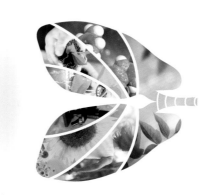

中国结核病防治生态图

健康促进

对象	措施	实施主体
适龄儿童	卡介苗接种	医疗机构
公众	健康生活方式 / 个人防护 / 健康体检	个人 / 个人 / 体检机构
重点人群	主动发现 / 感染筛查 / 预防性治疗	疾控机构 / 疾控和医疗机构 / 疾控和医疗机构
医疗机构	感染控制	医疗机构
聚集疫情	监测 / 处置	疾控机构 / 疾控和定点医院

患者关怀

对象	措施	实施主体
可疑症状者	问诊 / 推介转诊 / 实验室检查 / 影像学检查	医疗机构和基层 / 基层机构 / 医疗机构 / 医疗机构
疑似患者	报告 / 转诊 / 追踪	医疗机构和基层医疗机构 / 非定点医疗机构 / 疾控和基层
肺结核患者	诊断与报告 / 登记与治疗 / 服药管理	医疗机构 / 定点医院 / 疾控、定点医院和基层

全流程关怀服务

以患者为中心的"防、诊、治、管、教"

政策支持系统

支持主体	职责
卫生健康委	统筹协调
发展改革委	基础设施
财政部	经费投入
医保局	医疗保障
民政部	社会救助
扶贫办/红十字	贫困救助
食药总局	药品审批监管
工信部	药品试剂供应
教育部	学校防控
公安司法部	监管场所
农业农村部	人畜共患
质检总局	口岸监测
科技部	科研
广电总局	宣传
中医药局	中医治疗
社会组织	社会支持

工作机制 政府组织领导，部门各负其责、全社会共同参与

服务体系 疾控机构、医疗机构和基层医疗卫生机构分工明确协调配合

政策保障 政府投入为主、多渠道筹资，纳入社会发展规划

研究创新 基础研究和应用研究紧密结合，加快科技成果转化

中国结核病防治策略

以患者为中心的"防、诊、治、管、救"综合防治措施

预防

预防接种
新生儿卡介苗接种

预防性治疗
潜伏感染者预防性治疗

感染控制
环境感染控制
个人防护

预防性治疗对象：
1. 与病原学阳性患者密切接触的<5岁儿童潜伏感染者
2. 艾滋病病毒感染者及艾滋病患者中的潜伏感染者
3. 与活动性肺结核患者密切接触的学生等新近潜伏感染者

预防性治疗方案：
1. 单用异烟肼方案：每日1次6~9个月
2. 异烟肼、利福喷丁方案：每周2次3个月
3. 异烟肼、利福平方案：每日1次3个月
4. 单用利福平方案：每日1次4个月

早发现和早报告

患者发现

主动筛查
- 病原学阳性患者密切接触者
- 艾滋病病毒感染者及艾滋病患者
- 学校等重点场所

因症就诊
- 因症就诊
- 因症转诊追踪

登记报告
- 疑情报告
- 信息登记报告

1. 问诊及体格检查
2. 实验室检查
 • 传统检测
 • 分子生物学检测
3. 胸部影像学检查

1. 24小时内录入
2. 所有确诊病例均报告登记

早发现、早诊断、早报告

早治疗

利福平敏感
门诊治疗为主

利福平耐药
住院与门诊相结合

1. 异烟肼敏感：2HRZE/4HR
2. 异烟肼耐药：6-9RZELfx
3. 结核病胸膜炎：2HRZE(7-10)HRE

1. 长程治疗方案：
氟喹诺酮类敏感：6Lfx (Mfx) BdqLzd(Cs)Cfz/12Lfx (Mfx) Cfz
氟喹诺酮类耐药：6 Bdq Lzd Cfz Cs/14 Lzd Cfz Cs
2. 短程治疗方案：
4-6Lfx (Mfx) Bdq (Am) Cfz ZH (高剂量) Pto E/5 Lfx (Mfx) Cfz Z E
3. 治疗后效果评估

早期、联合、适量、规律、全程

全程管理和关怀

全程管理

1. 治疗前健康教育
2. 治疗过程管理
 • 住院管理
 • 门诊随访管理
 • 基层入户随访
 • 督导服药
3. 治疗后效果评估

全面关怀

1. 咨询服务
2. 心理咨询
3. 消除歧视
4. 同伴教育
5. 营养支持
6. 交通补助
7. 权益保障

全程管理和全面关怀

健康教育
预防接种、重点干预
全社会参与，分类指导，形式多样的宣教活动

培训督导
早发现、早诊断、早报告
问题导向，聚焦重点难点，有计划统筹开展

监控评价
早期、联合、适量、规律、全程
问题导向，聚焦重点难点，及时分析利用，指导结核病防控工作

研究创新
全程管理和全面关怀
基础研究和应用研究紧密结合，加快科技成果转化

中国结核病防治关键技术措施

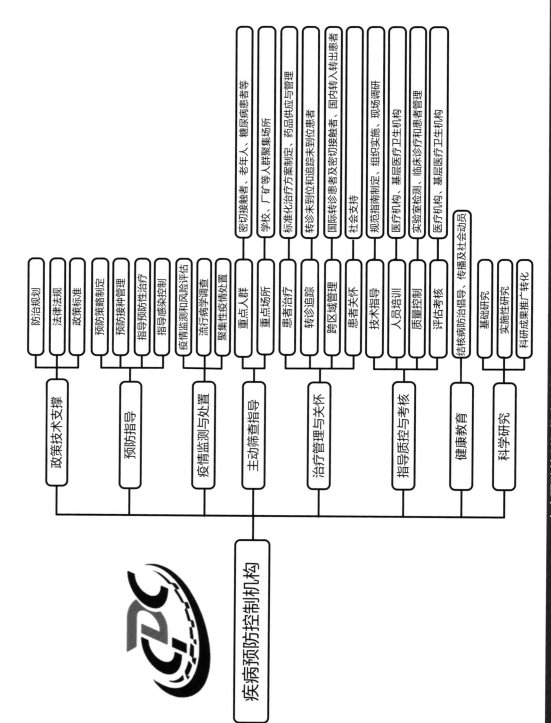

疾病预防控制机构

政策技术支撑
- 防治规划
- 法律法规
- 政策标准

预防指导
- 预防策略制定
- 预防接种管理
- 指导预防性治疗
- 指导感染控制

疫情监测与处置
- 疫情监测和风险评估
- 流行病学调查
- 聚集性疫情处置

主动筛查指导
- 重点人群 —— 密切接触者、老年人、糖尿病患者等
- 重点场所 —— 学校、厂矿等人群聚集场所

治疗管理与关怀
- 患者治疗 —— 标准化治疗方案制定、药品供应与管理
- 转诊追踪 —— 转诊未到位和追踪未到位患者
- 跨区域管理 —— 国际转诊患者及密切接触者、国内转入转出患者
- 患者关怀 —— 社会支持

指导质控与考核
- 技术指导 —— 规范指南制定、组织实施、现场调研
- 人员培训 —— 医疗机构、基层医疗卫生机构
- 质量控制 —— 实验室检测、临床诊疗和患者管理
- 评估考核 —— 医疗机构、基层医疗卫生机构

健康教育
- 结核病防治倡导、传播及社会动员

科学研究
- 基础研究
- 实施性研究
- 科研成果推广转化

疾病预防控制机构在结核病防治中的主要工作任务

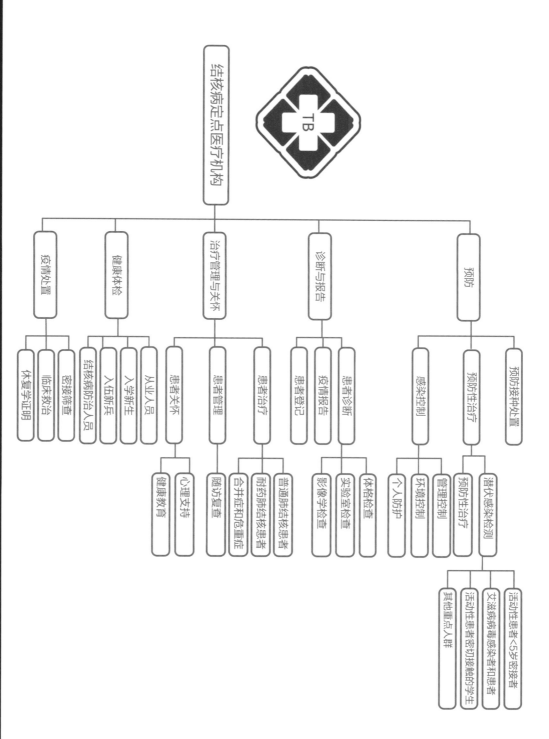

结核病定点医疗机构在结核病防治中的主要工作任务

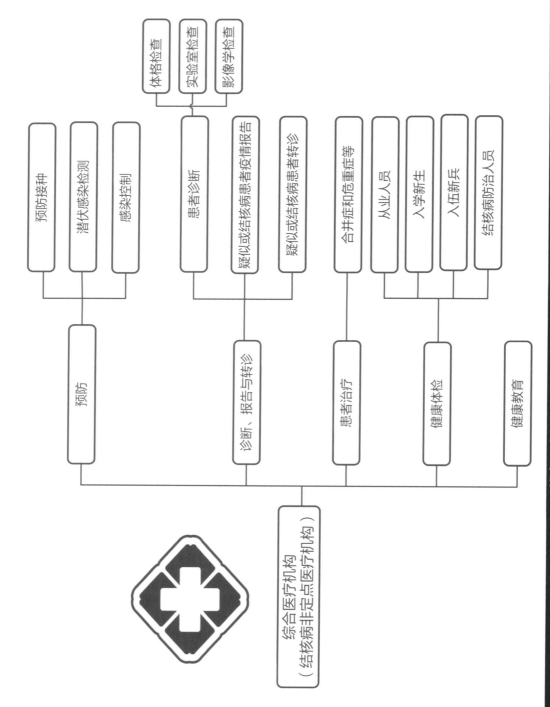

综合医疗机构在结核病防治中的主要工作任务

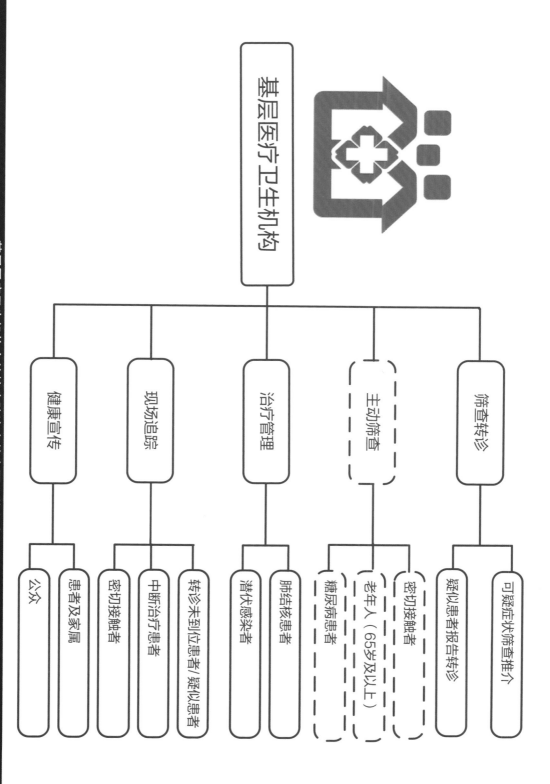

基层医疗卫生机构在结核病防治中的主要工作任务

基层医疗卫生机构

- 健康宣传
  - 公众
  - 患者及家属
- 现场追踪
  - 密切接触者
  - 中断治疗患者
  - 转诊未到位患者/疑似患者
- 治疗管理
  - 潜伏感染者
  - 肺结核患者
- 主动筛查
  - 糖尿病患者
  - 老年人（65岁及以上）
  - 密切接触者
- 筛查转诊
  - 疑似患者报告转诊
  - 可疑症状筛查推介

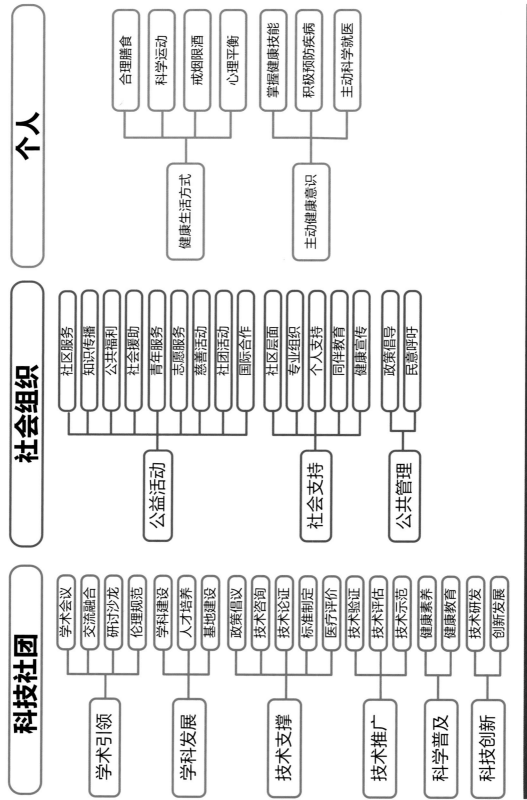

个人

健康生活方式
- 合理膳食
- 科学运动
- 戒烟限酒
- 心理平衡

主动健康意识
- 掌握健康技能
- 积极预防疾病
- 主动科学就医

社会组织

公益活动
- 社区服务
- 知识传播
- 公共福利
- 社会援助
- 青年服务
- 志愿服务
- 慈善活动
- 社团活动
- 国际合作

社会支持
- 社区层面
- 专业组织
- 个人支持
- 同伴教育
- 健康宣传

公共管理
- 政策倡导
- 民意呼吁

科技社团

学术引领
- 学术会议
- 交流融合
- 研讨沙龙
- 伦理规范

学科发展
- 学科建设
- 人才培养
- 基地建设

技术支撑
- 政策倡议
- 技术咨询
- 技术论证
- 标准制定
- 医疗评价

技术推广
- 技术验证
- 技术评估
- 技术示范

科学普及
- 健康素养
- 健康教育

科技创新
- 技术研发
- 创新发展

科技社团、社会组织和个人在结核病防治中的主要工作任务

结核病实验室质量管理

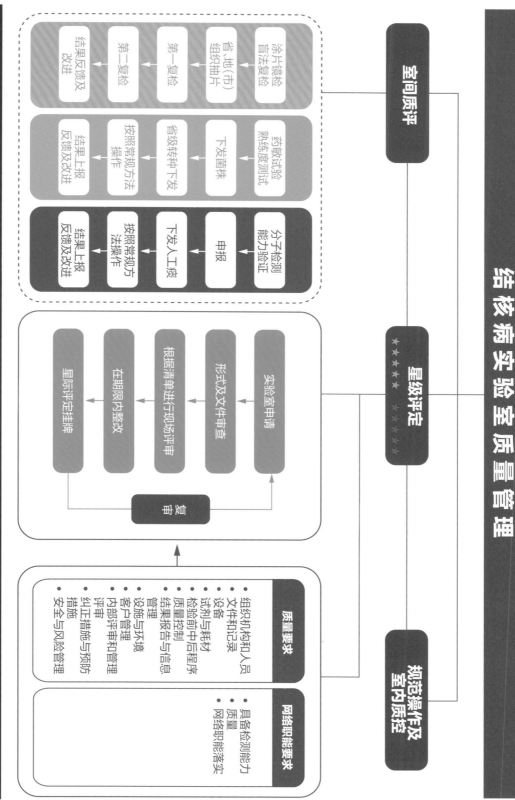

室间质评

星级评定
★★★★
★★★★★
★★★★★★

规范操作及室内质控

涂片镜检管法复检
省，地（市）组织抽片
第一复检
第二复检
结果反馈及改进

药敏试验熟练度测试
下发菌株
省级特种下发
按照常规方法操作
结果上报反馈及改进

分子检测熟练能力验证
申报
下发人工浆
按照常规方法操作
结果上报反馈及改进

实验室申请
形式及文件审查
根据清单进行现场评审
在期限内整改
星际评定挂牌

复审

质量要求
• 组织机构和人员
• 文件和记录
• 设备
• 试剂与耗材
• 检验前中后程序
• 质量控制
• 结果报告与信息管理
• 设施与环境
• 客户管理
• 内部评审和管理评审
• 纠正措施与预防措施
• 安全与风险管理

网络职能要求
• 具备检测能力
• 质量
• 网络职能落实

中国结核病防治生态图集

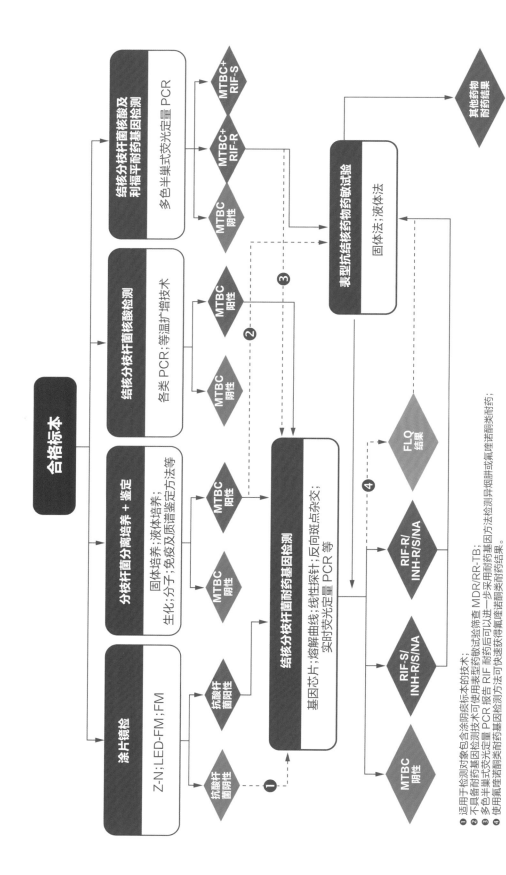

结核病病原学检测方法及临床应用

❶ 适用于检测对象包含阴痰标本的技术；
❷ 不具备耐药基因检测技术可使用表型药敏检测筛查 MDR/RR-TB；
❸ 多色半巢式荧光定量 PCR 报告 RIF 耐药后可以进一步采用耐药基因方法检测异烟肼或喹诺酮类耐药；
❹ 使用氟喹诺酮类耐药基因检测方法可快速获得喹诺酮类氟喹诺酮类耐药结果。

10

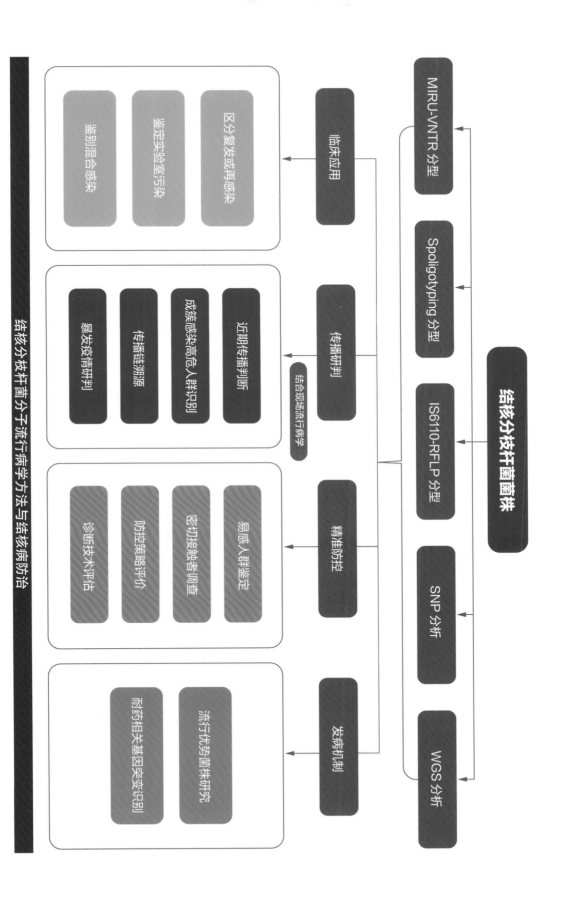

结核分枝杆菌菌株

- MIRU-VNTR 分型
- Spoligotyping 分型
- IS6110-RFLP 分型
- SNP 分析
- WGS 分析

临床应用
- 区分复发或再感染
- 鉴定实验室污染
- 鉴别混合感染

传播研判（结合现场流行病学）
- 近期传播判断
- 成簇感染高危人群识别
- 传播链溯源
- 暴发疫情研判

精准防控
- 易感人群鉴定
- 密切接触者调查
- 防控策略评价
- 诊断技术评估

发病机制
- 流行优势菌株研究
- 耐药相关基因突变识别

结核分枝杆菌分子流行病学方法与结核病防治

中国结核病防治生态图集

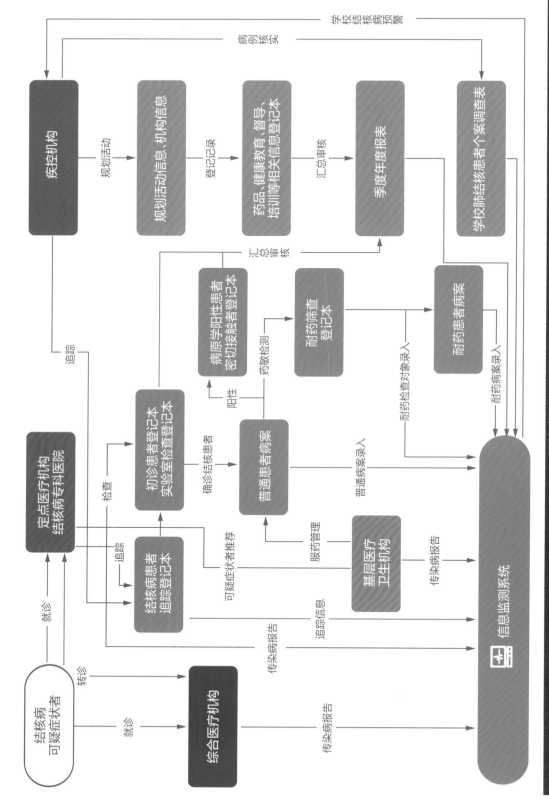

结核病信息监测流程

结核病信息监测

工作领域	监测内容	规划登记表本卡册	信息监测系统
主动筛查	病原学阳性患者接触者筛查信息；学校患者接触者筛查信息；老年人筛查信息；糖尿病患者筛查信息	病原学阳性肺结核患者密切接触者筛查登记录；学校肺结核患者密切接触者症状筛查一览表；老年人肺结核可疑症状筛查和推介表；糖尿病患者肺结核可疑症状筛查和推介表	阳性肺结核患者密切接触者检查情况；学校肺结核患者密切接触者检查情况；老年人肺结核筛查情况；糖尿病患者肺结核筛查情况
预防性治疗	HIV感染者/AIDS患者开展结核检查信息；重点人群预防性服药信息	结核病预防性治疗登记本	HIV感染者/AIDS患者开展结核病检查情况；预防性治疗情况
实验室检查	患者诊断和随访过程中实验室检查信息	痰涂片检查登记本；分枝杆菌培养检查登记本；结核分枝杆菌核酸检测登记本；药物敏感性试验登记本；结核分枝杆菌耐药相关基因检测登记本	结核病检查对象信息；耐药检查对象信息；耐药结核病患者病案
患者诊断	结核门诊诊断信息	初诊患者登记本	初诊患者检查情况
疫情报告	疑似或确诊患者填报卡	传染病报告卡	报告卡管理
转诊追踪	未到位患者的收治信息；耐药患者的追踪信息	肺结核患者或疑似肺结核患者追踪情况登记本；利福平耐药肺结核患者追踪管理登记本	追踪信息管理
患者登记	结核病患者诊断和治疗转归信息；耐多药患者诊断和治疗归信息	耐药患者门诊病案；结核病患者登记本；利福平耐药结核病患者病案	耐药检查对象信息；结核病患者病案；耐药结核病患者病案
治疗管理	利福平耐药患者服药信息；肺结核患者服药信息；跨区域管理；患者取药信息	肺结核患者服药记录卡；利福平耐药肺结核患者服药记录卡	药品使用信息
疫情处置	学校疫情信息	抗结核药品不良反应报告表；患者转入转出信息	转入转出信息
规划活动	痰涂片复查复检；TB/HIV双重感染患者治疗信息；本级财政对结核病防治投入情况；开展健康教育活动；开展培训；督导工作；结核病防治机构信息	学校肺结核报卡信息核查表	学校结核病单病例预警系统；痰涂片法复检结果；TB/HIV双重感染患者治疗情况；结核病防治专项投入情况；开展健康教育活动投入情况；培训工作开展情况；督导情况；结核病防治机构信息

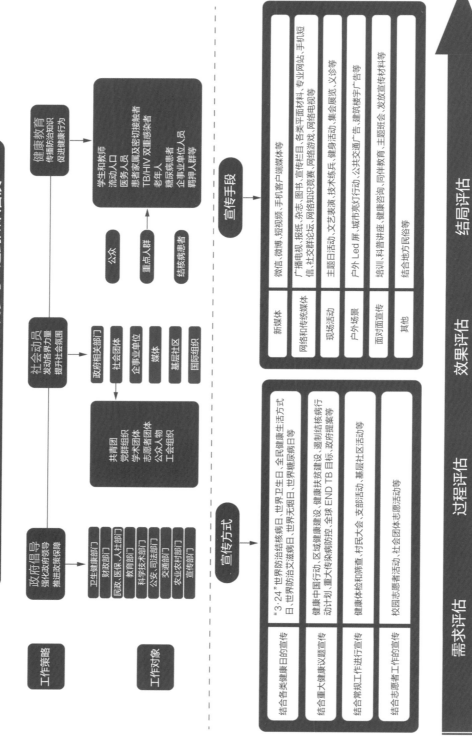

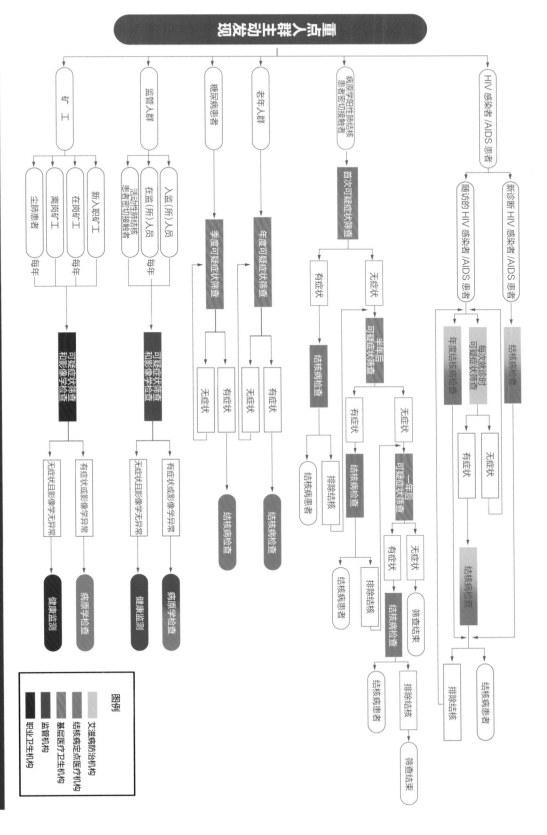

重点人群主动发现

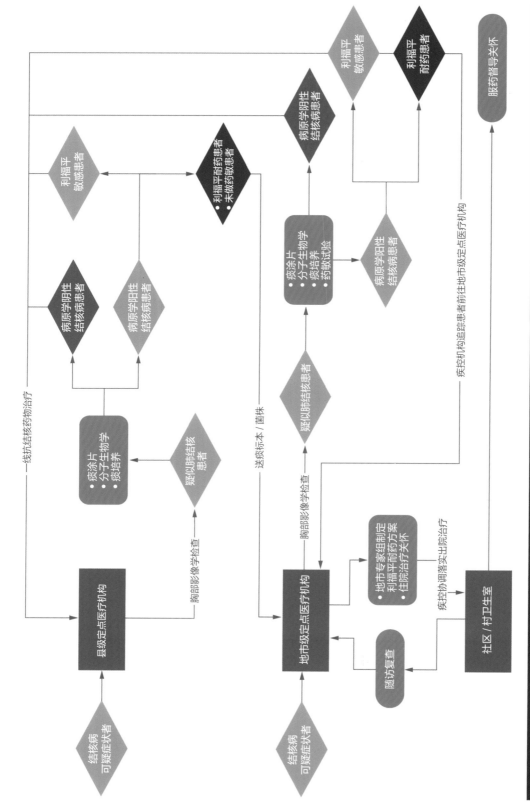

耐药结核病诊断治疗管理

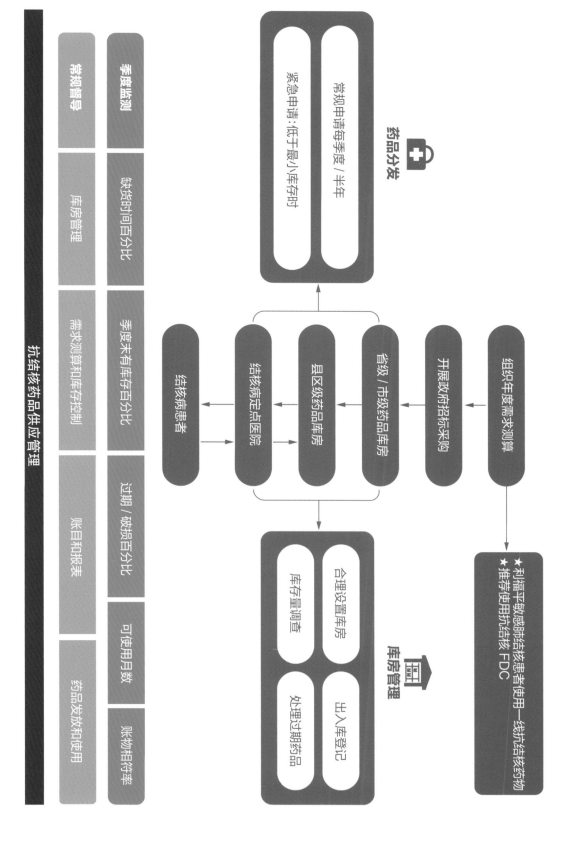

药品分发

常规申请每季度/半年

紧急申请：低于最小库存时

组织年度需求测算

开展政府招标采购

省级/市级药品库房

县区级药品库房

结核病定点医院

结核病患者

★ 利福平敏感肺结核患者使用一线抗结核药物
★ 推荐使用抗结核 FDC

库房管理

合理设置库房

库存量调查

出入库登记

处理过期药品

抗结核药品供应管理

季度监测

缺货时间百分比

季度末有库存百分比

过期/破损百分比

可使用月数

账物相符率

常规督导

库房管理

需求测算和库存控制

账目和报表

药品发放和使用

中国结核病防治生态图集

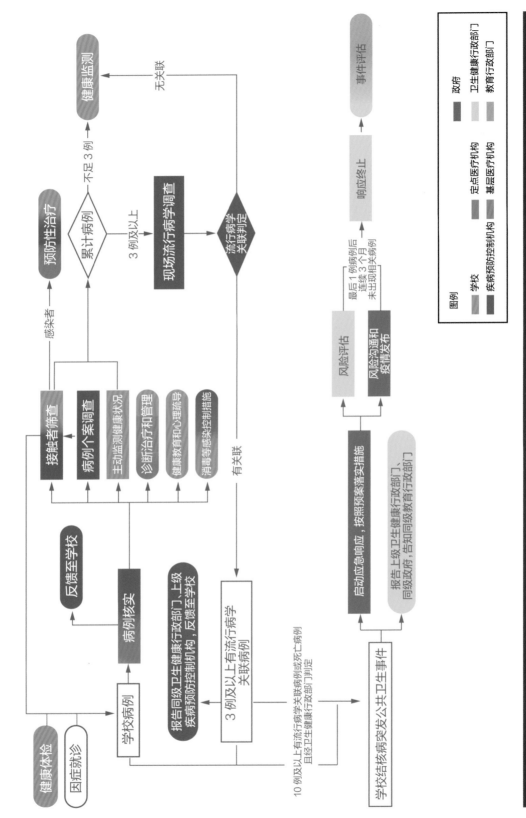

学校结核病疫情处置

结核感染控制

三防	疾病预防控制机构	定点医疗机构	基层医疗卫生机构	社区与家庭
组织管理	本地区感染控制规划 管理制度与标准操作程序 经费保障与人才培养 宣传与促进 开展实施性研究 监控与评价	感染控制委员会 感染控制工作计划 健康促进与教育 机构感染控制风险评估 优化建筑布局和设置 人员培训 医务人员健康监测	感染控制工作计划 接受培训 健康监测	社区健康宣传
行政控制	没有结核门诊： 预检分诊 分诊就诊 患者佩戴外科口罩 标准化预防 缩短停留时间，早诊早治 没有结核实验室： 专人送检 出入管理限制	预检分诊 患者分类就诊和安置 标准化预防 缩短建筑停留时间，早诊早治 患者佩戴外科口罩	预检分诊 转诊推荐 标准化预防	分室居住
环境控制	生物安全设施设备 通风系统使用与维护 紫外线杀菌装置使用与维护	通风系统使用与维护 紫外线杀菌装置使用与维护	通风与消毒	居室通风 痰液等消毒处理
呼吸防护	实验室人员佩戴医用防护口罩	基于风险评估，医护人员佩戴医用防护口罩	医务人员与肺结核患者/疑似患者接触时，佩戴医用防护口罩	与患者接触时尽量佩戴医用防护口罩

结核感染控制

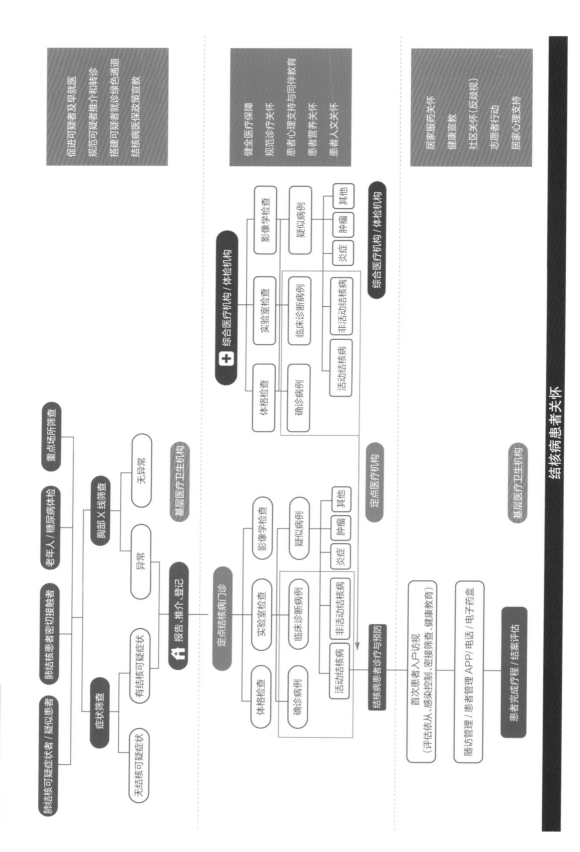

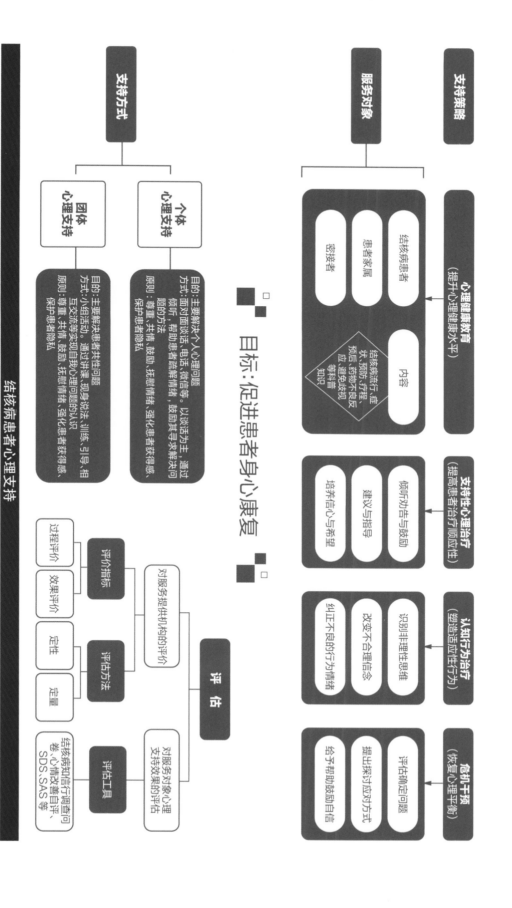

结核病患者心理支持

目标：促进患者身心康复

支持策略

心理健康教育（提升心理健康水平）

内容：结核病流行现状、预后、药物不良反应、避免传染等科普知识

支持性心理治疗（提高患者治疗顺应性）
- 倾听劝告与鼓励
- 建议与指导
- 培养信心与希望

认知行为治疗（塑造适应性行为）
- 识别非理性思维
- 改变不合理信念
- 纠正不良的行为情绪

危机干预（恢复心理平衡）
- 评估确定问题
- 提出探讨应对方式
- 给予帮助和鼓励自信

服务对象
- 结核病患者
- 患者家属
- 密接者

支持方式

个体心理支持
方式：主要解决个人心理问题
方式：面对面谈话、电话、微信等，以谈话为主，通过倾听，帮助患者疏解情绪，鼓励其寻求解决问题的方法
原则：尊重、共情，鼓励患者自我现身说法，强化患者获得感，保护患者隐私

团体心理支持
目的：主要解决患者共性心理问题
方式：小组活动，通过讲课、现身说法、训练、引导、相互交流等实现身心的认识
原则：尊重，共情，鼓励自我现身说法，强化患者获得感，保护患者隐私

评估

对服务提供机构的评价

评价指标
- 过程评价
- 效果评价

评估方法
- 定性
- 定量

对服务对象心理支持效果的评估

评估工具
结核病知信行调查问卷、心情自评、SDS、SAS等

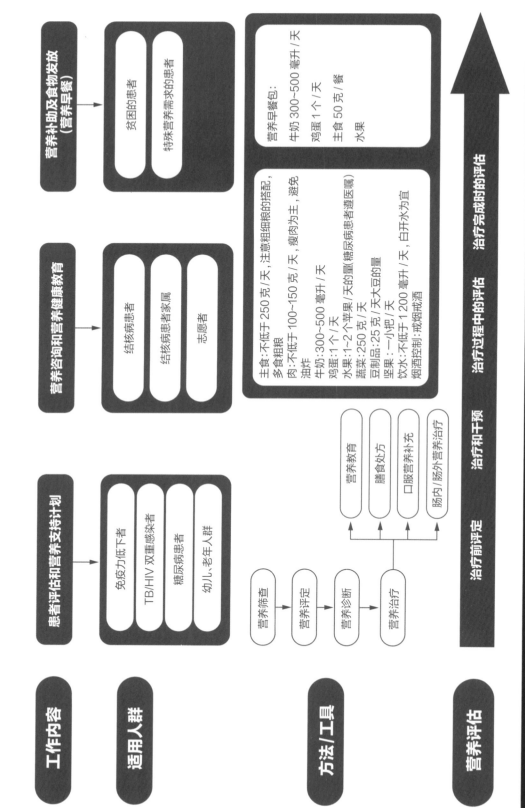

中国结核病防治生态图集

结核病患者营养支持

| 工作内容 | 患者评估和营养支持计划 | 营养咨询和营养健康教育 | 营养补助及食物发放（营养早餐） |

适用人群

患者评估和营养支持计划：
- 免疫力低下者
- TB/HIV 双重感染者
- 糖尿病患者
- 幼儿、老年人群

营养咨询和营养健康教育：
- 结核病患者
- 结核病患者家属
- 志愿者

营养补助及食物发放（营养早餐）：
- 贫困的患者
- 特殊营养需求的患者

方法/工具

营养筛查 → 营养评定 → 营养诊断 → 营养治疗

- 营养教育
- 膳食处方
- 口服营养补充
- 肠内/肠外营养治疗

主食：不低于 250 克/天，注意粗细粮的搭配，多食粗粮
肉：不低于 100~150 克/天，瘦肉为主，避免油炸
牛奶：300~500 毫升/天
鸡蛋：1 个/天
水果：1~2 个苹果/天（糖尿病患者遵医嘱的量）
蔬菜：250 克/天
豆制品：25 克/天大大豆的量
坚果：一小把/天
饮水：不低于 1 200 毫升/天，白开水为宜
烟酒控制：戒烟戒酒

营养早餐包：
牛奶 300~500 毫升/天
鸡蛋 1 个/天
主食 50 克/餐
水果

营养评估

治疗前评定 → 治疗过程中的评估 → 治疗完成时的评估

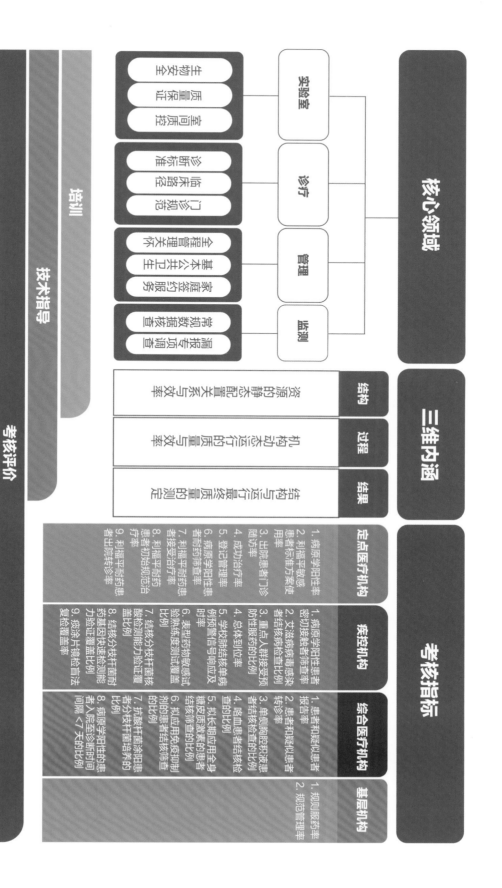

China's tuberculosis control and prevention ecosystem

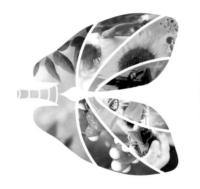

Overall goal: to reduce the incidence and death of tuberculosis and the economic burden of patients

Prevention

Objects	Measures	Implementation subjects
Age-appropriate children	BCG vaccination	Medical institutions
Public	Healthy lifestyle	Individuals
	Personal protection	Individuals
	Health examination	Health examination institutions
Key population	Active discovery	CDCs and medical institutions
	Infection screening	CDCs and medical institutions
	Preventive treatment	Centers for disease control and prevention
Medical institutions	Infection control	Medical institutions
Clustered epidemic	Monitoring	CDCs
	Response	CDCs and designated hospitals

Health promotion

Diagnosis, treatment and management

Objects	Measures	Implementation subjects
People with TB symptoms	Inquiry	Medical institutions primary health institutions
	Referral	Primary health institutions
	Laboratory examination	Medical institutions
	Imaging examination	Medical institutions
Presumptive TB patients	Case notificaiton	CDCs and primary health institutions
	Referral	Non-designated medical institutions
	Tracing	Medical institutions
TB patients	Diagnosis and case notification	Designated hospitals
	Registration and treatment	Medical institutions
	Medication management	CDCs, designated hospitals and primary health institutions

Patient care

Multi-sectoral cooperation

Duties	Support subjects
Overall coordination	Health Commission
Infrastructure	Development and Reform Commission
Funding	Ministry of Finance
Medical insurance	Medical Insurance Bureau
Social assistance	Ministry of Civil Affairs
Poverty relief	Poverty Alleviation Office/Red Cross
Drug approval and supervision	Food and Drug Administration
Drug/reagent supply	Ministry of Industry and Information Technology
School prevention and control	Ministry of Education
Prisons and supervision sites	Ministry of Public Security/Justice
Zoonotic Diseases	Ministry of Agriculture and Rural Affairs
International port supervision	Administration of Quality Supervision
Research	Ministry of Science and Technology
Publicizing	State Administration of Radio, Film and Television
Chinese traditional medicine	Chinese Medicine Bureau
Social support	Non-government organizations

Patient-centered "prevention, diagnosis, treatment, management and education" whole-process care service

Policy Support System

Working Mechanism
Under government's leadership, different sections take their respective responsibilities, and the whole society participates

service system
With clear division of labor, CDCs, medical institutions and primary health institutions closely collaborated

Policy assurance
Multi-channel fund-raising dominated by governmental investment, incorporated into the social development plan

Research and innovation
Close integration of basic research and applied research to accelerate the transformation of scientific and technological achievements

Tuberculosis control and prevention strategy

China's tuberculosis control and prevention ecosystem

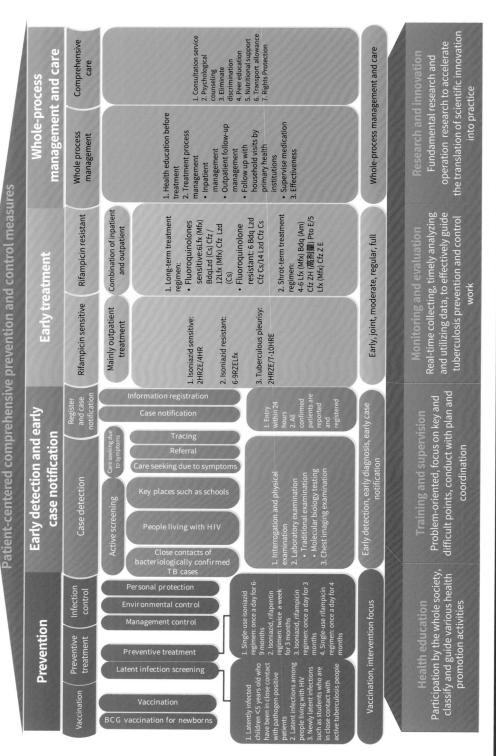

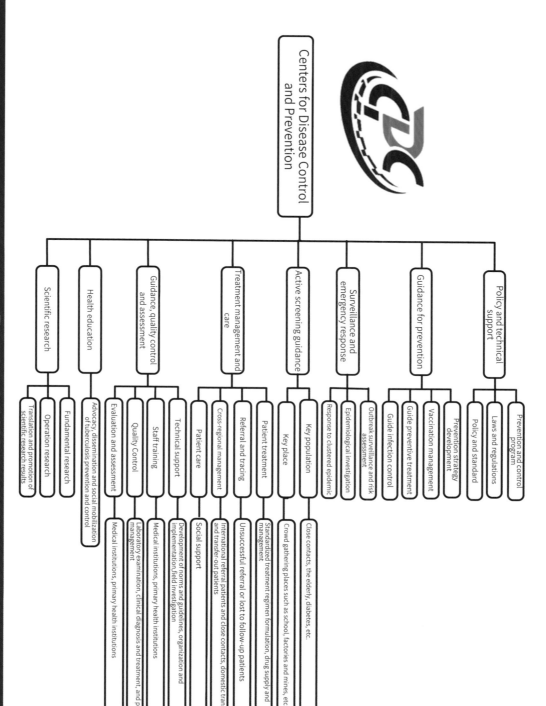

Centers for Disease Control and Prevention

Policy and technical support
- Prevention and control program
- Laws and regulations
- Policy and standard

Guidance for prevention
- Prevention strategy development
- Vaccination management
- Guide preventive treatment
- Guide infection control

Surveillance and emergency response
- Outbreak surveillance and risk assessment
- Epidemiological investigation
- Response to clustered epidemic

Active screening guidance
- Key population
  - Close contacts, the elderly, diabetes, etc.
  - Crowd gathering places such as school, factories and mines, etc.
- Key place

Treatment management and care
- Patient treatment
  - Standardized treatment regimen formulation, drug supply and management
- Referral and tracing
  - Unsuccessful referral or lost to follow-up patients
  - International referral patients and close contacts, domestic transfer-in and transfer-out patients
- Cross-regional management
- Patient care
  - Social support
  - Development of norms and guidelines, organization and implementation, field investigation

Guidance, quality control and assessment
- Technical support
  - Medical institutions, primary health institutions
- Staff training
  - Laboratory examination, clinical diagnosis and treatment, and patient management
- Quality Control
  - Medical institutions, primary health institutions
- Evaluation and assessment
  - Medical institutions, primary health institutions

Health education
- Advocacy, dissemination and social mobilization of tuberculosis prevention and control

Scientific research
- Fundamental research
- Operation research
- Translation and promotion of scientific research results

China's tuberculosis control and prevention ecosystem

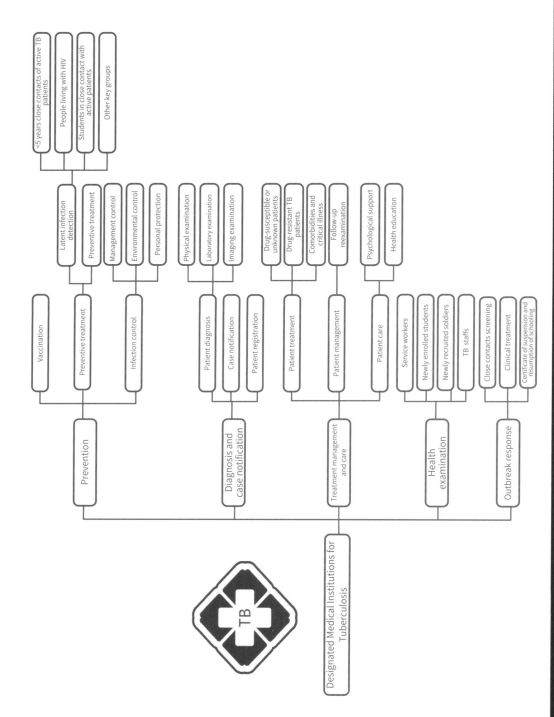

The main task of TB designated medical institutions for tuberculosis

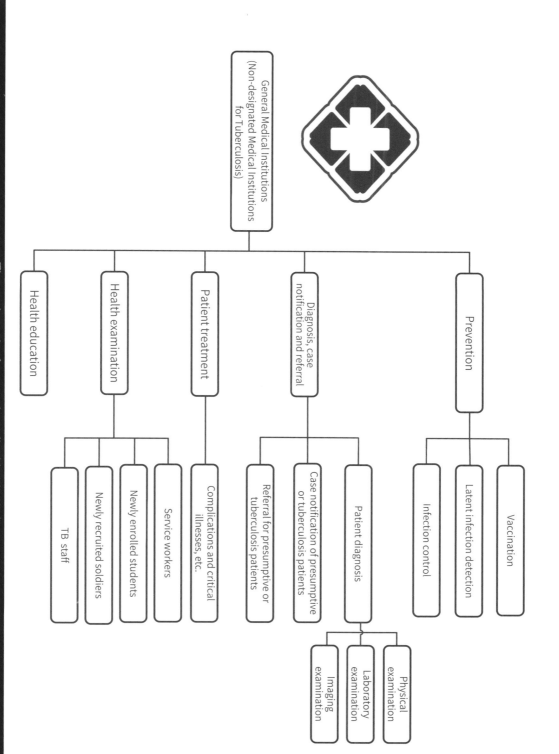

The main task of general medical institutions

General Medical Institutions (Non-designated Medical Institutions for Tuberculosis)

- Health education
- Health examination
  - TB staff
  - Newly recruited soldiers
  - Newly enrolled students
  - Service workers
- Patient treatment
  - Complications and critical illnesses, etc.
- Diagnosis, case notification and referral
  - Referral for presumptive or tuberculosis patients
  - Case notification of presumptive or tuberculosis patients
  - Patient diagnosis
    - Imaging examination
    - Laboratory examination
    - Physical examination
- Prevention
  - Infection control
  - Latent infection detection
  - Vaccination

China's tuberculosis control and prevention ecosystem

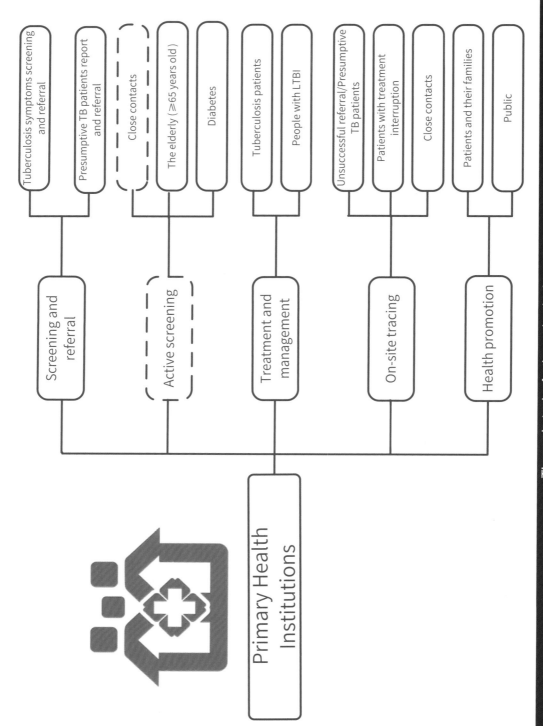

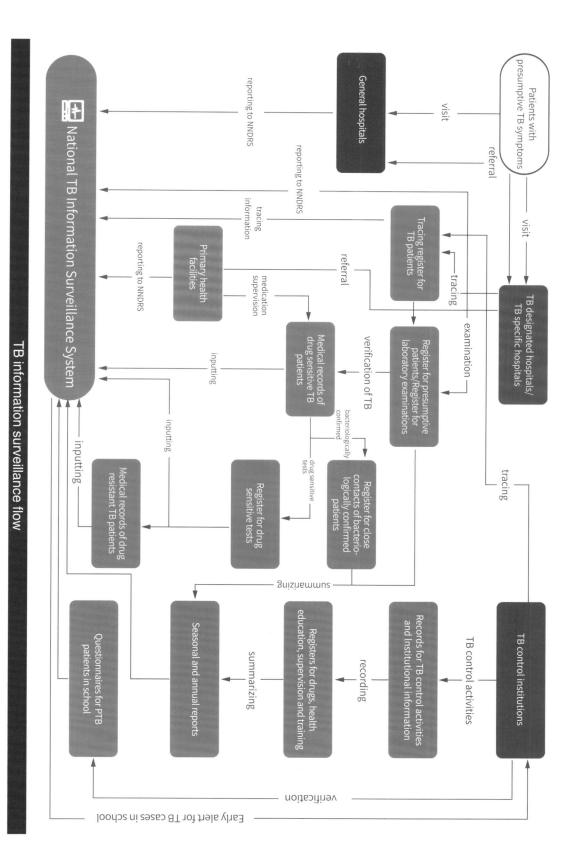

China's tuberculosis control and prevention ecosystem

TB information surveillance flow

China's tuberculosis control and prevention ecosystem

Domains

- Active screening
- TB preventive treatment
- Laboratory examinations
- Patients diagnosis
- Reporting
- Referral and tracing
- Notification
- Treatment management
- Cluster management
- NTP activities

Surveillance content

- Screening results among close contacts of bacteriologically confirmed patients
- Screening results among contacts of school patients
- Screening results among elder patients
- Screening results among diabetes
- TB examination results among HIV/AIDS
- TPT among key populations
- Laboratory examinations during patients diagnosis and follow-up
- Diagnosis results in TB outpatient departments
- Reporting cards for presumptive or diagnosed TB patients
- Diagnosis results of arrived patients
- Tracing results of patients not arriving
- Tracing results of drug resistant patients
- Diagnosis and treatment outcomes of TB patients
- Drug susceptibility test results
- Diagnosis and treatment information for drug resistant patients
- Medication records for PTB patients
- Medication records for RR-TB patients
- Cross-areas management
- Patients' drug collection information
- Clusters in school
- Blind review results for sputum smear examinations
- Treatment outcomes for TB/HIV patients
- Local imbursement in TB control
- Health education activities
- Training activities
- Supervision activities
- Information of TB control institutions

Cards, records, lists and registers

- Register for screening results among close contacts of bacteriologically confirmed patients
- List for screening results among contacts of school PTB patients
- Register for referral and screening results among elders with PTB symptoms
- Register for referral and screening results among diabetes
- Register for TB preventive treatment
- Register for sputum smear examinations
- Register for Mycobacterium cultures
- Register for MTB nucleic acid tests
- Register for drug susceptibility tests
- Register for MTB drug resistance related genes tests
- Register for presumptive patients
- Infectious disease reporting cards
- Register for tracing results of presumptive or diagnosed PTB patients
- Register for tracing and management of RR-TB patients
- Medical records for TB outpatients
- Register for drug susceptibility tests
- Medical records for RR-TB patients
- Medication taken records for PTB patients
- Medication taken records for RR-TB patients
- Records for patients transfer-in and transfer-out information
- Register for anti-TB drugs delivery
- Checklist for PTB reporting cards in school

Information surveillance system modules

- Screening results among close contacts of bacteriologically confirmed patients
- Screening results among contacts of school PTB patients
- TB screening results among elder patients
- TB screening results among diabetes
- HIV/AIDS TB examination results among HIV/AIDS
- Results of TB preventive treatment
- Medical records for TB patients
- Records for drug sensitivity tests
- Medical records for drug resistant TB patients
- Examination results for presumptive patients
- Reporting cards management
- Tracing information management
- Records for drug sensitivity tests
- Medical records for TB patients
- Records for drug sensitivity tests
- Medical records for drug resistant TB patients
- Medical records for TB patients
- Medical records for drug resistant TB patients
- Transfer-in and transfer-out management
- Drug inventory management
- Single case alert system for school TB patient
- Blind review results for sputum smear examinations
- Treatment outcomes for TB/HIV patients
- Financial imbursement in TB control
- Health education activities management
- Training activities management
- Supervision activities management
- Management of TB control institutions information

TB information surveillance

36

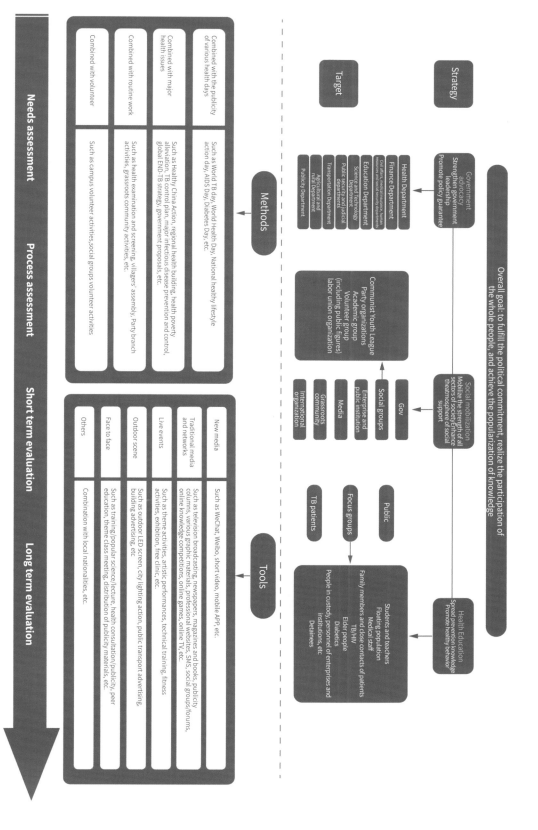

China's tuberculosis control and prevention ecosystem

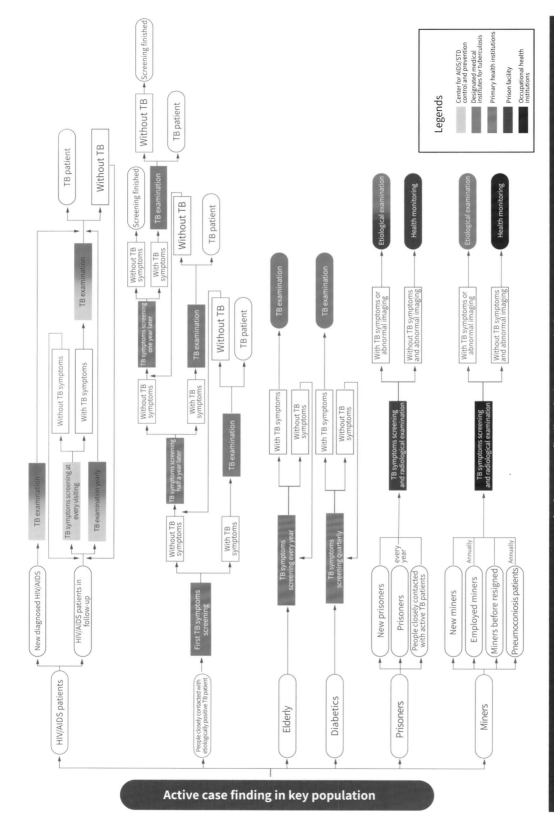

Active case finding in key population

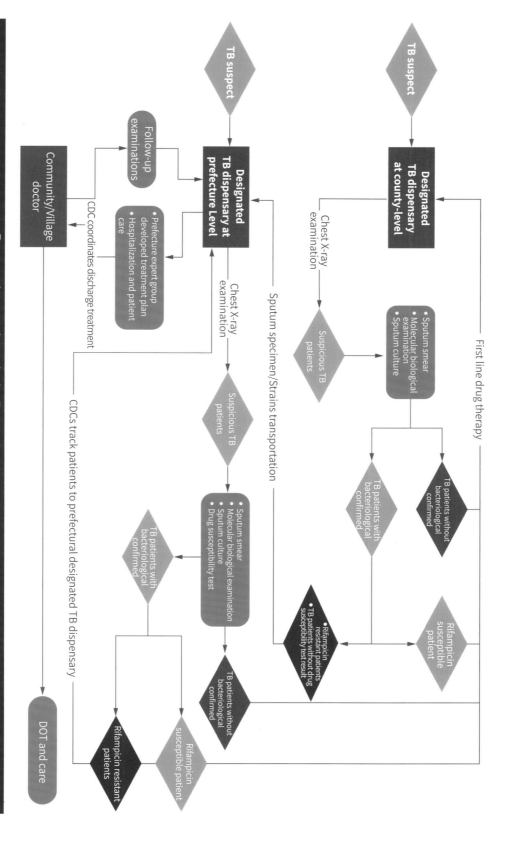

Drug-resistant tuberculosis diagnosis treatment management

China's tuberculosis control and prevention ecosystem

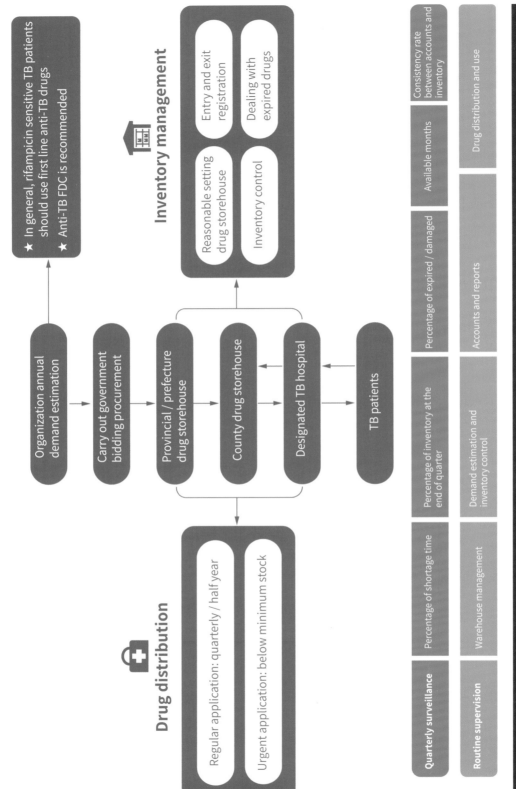

★ In general, rifampicin sensitive TB patients should use first line anti-TB drugs
★ Anti-TB FDC is recommended

Inventory management

| Reasonable setting drug storehouse | Entry and exit registration |
| Inventory control | Dealing with expired drugs |

Organization annual demand estimation

Carry out government bidding procurement

Provincial / prefecture drug storehouse

County drug storehouse

Designated TB hospital

TB patients

Drug distribution

Regular application: quarterly / half year

Urgent application: below minimum stock

| Quarterly surveillance | Percentage of shortage time | Percentage of inventory at the end of quarter | Percentage of expired / damaged | Available months | Consistency rate between accounts and inventory |
| Routine supervision | Warehouse management | Demand estimation and inventory control | Accounts and reports | Drug distribution and use | |

Anti-TB drugs supply and management

China's tuberculosis control and prevention ecosystem

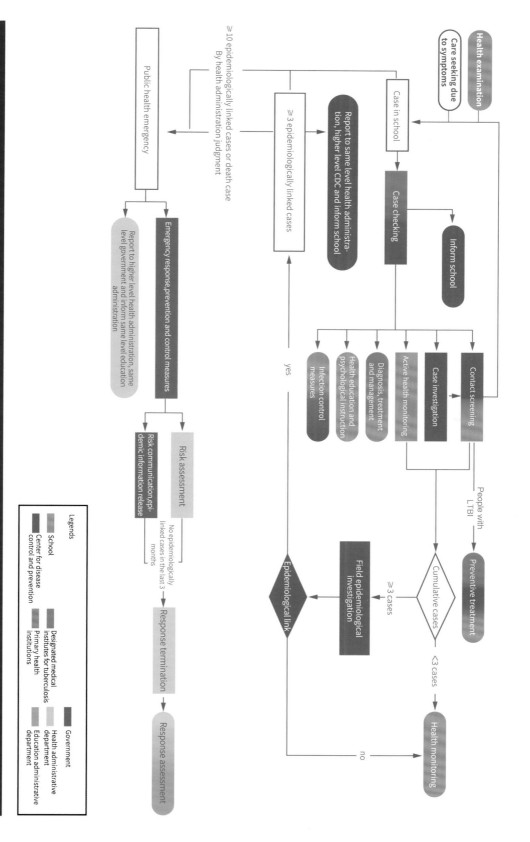

TB disposal in schools

41

China's tuberculosis control and prevention ecosystem

Tuberculosis Infection Control

	Centers for Diseases Control and Prevention	Designated Medical Institutions for Tuberculosis	Primary Health Institutions	Communities and Families
Managerial activities	Local infection control programme Management regulations and standard operating procedure Funding guarantee and human resources training Health education and promotion Implementation research Monitoring and evaluation	Infection Control Committee Infection control work plan Health education and promotion Infection control risk evaluation of the facilities Optimize building layout and settings Staff training Health surveillance of health-care workers	Infection Control Committee Receive trainingHealth surveillance	Health education
Administrative controls	If with TB outpatients: Pre-inspection and triage Separate visits Patients wear surgical masks Standard precaution Minimize stay time, early diagnosis and early treatment If with TB laboratory: Sputum delivery by dedicated worker Restricted access	Pre-inspection and triage Separate visits and management Standard precaution Minimize stay time, early diagnosis and early treatment Patients wear surgical masks	Pre-inspection and triage Suspected patient referral Standard precaution	Living in separate rooms
Environmental controls	Biosafety facilities and equipment Using and maintenance of ventilation systems Using and maintenance of UVGI fixtures	Using and maintenance of ventilation systems Using and maintenance of UVGI fixtures	Ventilation and disinfection	Room ventilation Disinfection of sputum
Respiratory protection	Laboratory staff wear medical protective respirators	Based on risk evaluation, health-care workers wear medical protective respirators	Health-care workers wear medical protective respirators, when in contact with TB patients of suspected patients	Wear medical protective respirators as much as possible, when in contact with TB patients

Tuberculosis infection control

China's tuberculosis control and prevention ecosystem

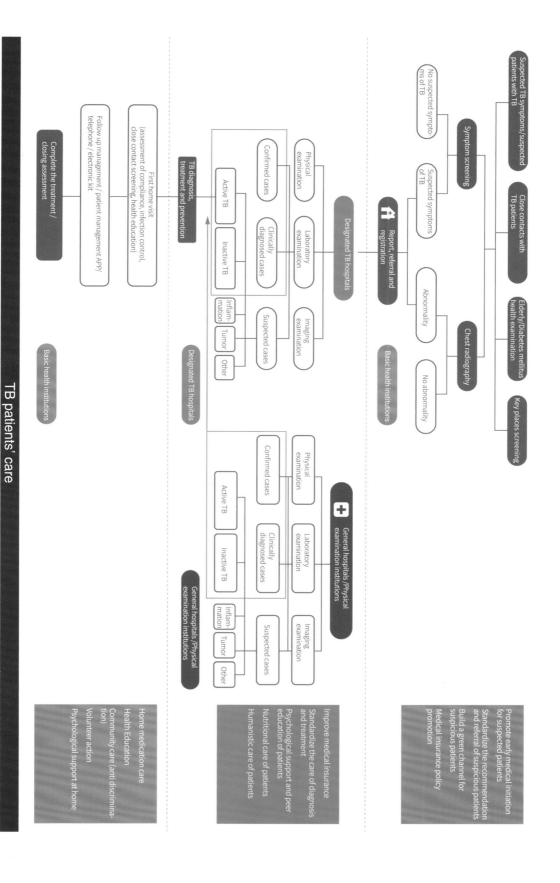

TB patients' care

Suspected TB symptoms/suspected patients with TB

No suspected symptoms of TB

Suspected symptoms of TB

Symptom screening

Close contacts with TB patients

Elderly/Diabetes mellitus health examination

Key places screening

Report, referral and registration

Abnormality

No abnormality

Chest radiography

Basic health institutions

Promote early medical initiation for suspected patients
Standardize the recommendation and referral of suspicious patients
Build a green channel for suspicious patients
Medical insurance policy promotion

Designated TB hospitals

Physical examination
Laboratory examination
Imaging examination

Confirmed cases
Clinically diagnosed cases
Suspected cases

Active TB
Inactive TB

Inflam-mation
Tumor
Other

Designated TB hospitals

Improve medical insurance
Standardize the care of diagnosis and treatment
Psychological support and peer education of patients
Nutritional care of patients
Humanistic care of patients

General hospitals /Physical examination institutions

Physical examination
Laboratory examination
Imaging examination

Confirmed cases
Clinically diagnosed cases
Suspected cases

Active TB
Inactive TB

Inflam-mation
Tumor
Other

General hospitals /Physical examination institutions

TB diagnosis, treatment and prevention

First home visit
(assessment of compliance, infection control, close contact screening, health education)

Follow up management / patient management APP/ telephone / electronic kit

Complete the treatment / closing assessment

Basic health institutions

Home medication care
Health Education
Community care (anti discrimina-tion)
Volunteer action
Psychological support at home

43

China's tuberculosis control and prevention ecosystem

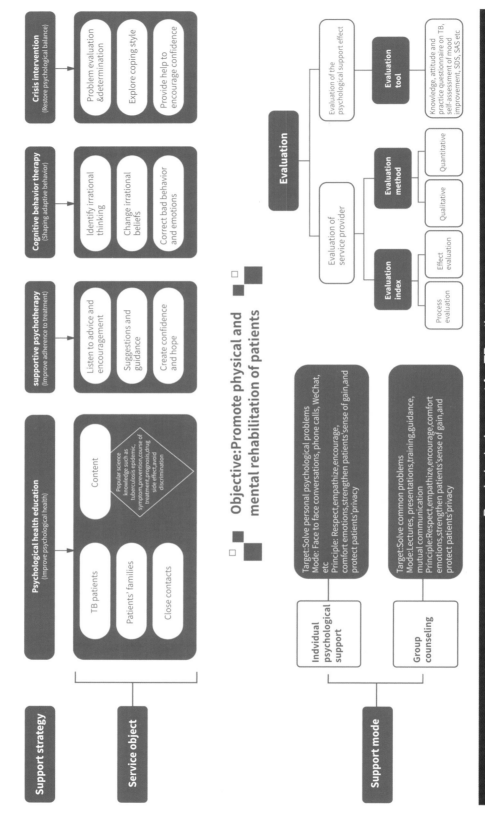

Support strategy

Psychological health education
(Improve psychological health)

Content

Popular science knowledge such as tuberculosis epidemic, symptom,prevention,course of treatment,prognosis,drug side effect,avoid discrimination

TB patients

Patients' families

Close contacts

supportive psychotherapy
(Improve adherence to treatment)

Listen to advice and encouragement

Suggestions and guidance

Create confidence and hope

Cognitive behavior therapy
(Shaping adaptive behavior)

Identify irrational thinking

Change irrational beliefs

Correct bad behavior and emotions

Crisis intervention
(Restore psychological balance)

Problem evaluation &determination

Explore coping style

Provide help to encourage confidence

Service object

□
■
■
Objective:Promote physical and mental rehabilitation of patients
□
■

Support mode

Individual psychological support

Target:Solve personal psychological problems
Mode: Face to face conversations, phone calls, WeChat, etc
Principle: Respect,empathize,encourage, comfort emotions,strengthen patients'sense of gain,and protect patients'privacy

Group counseling

Target:Solve common problems
Mode: Lectures, presentations,training,guidance, mutual communication
Principle:Respect,empathize,encourage,comfort emotions,strengthen patients'sense of gain,and protect patients'privacy

Evaluation

Evaluation of service provider

Evaluation index

Process evaluation

Effect evaluation

Evaluation method

Qualitative

Quantitative

Evaluation of the psychological support effect

Evaluation tool

Knowledge, attitude and practice questionnaire on TB, self-assessment of mood improvement, SDS, SAS etc

Psychological support for TB patients

China's tuberculosis control and prevention ecosystem

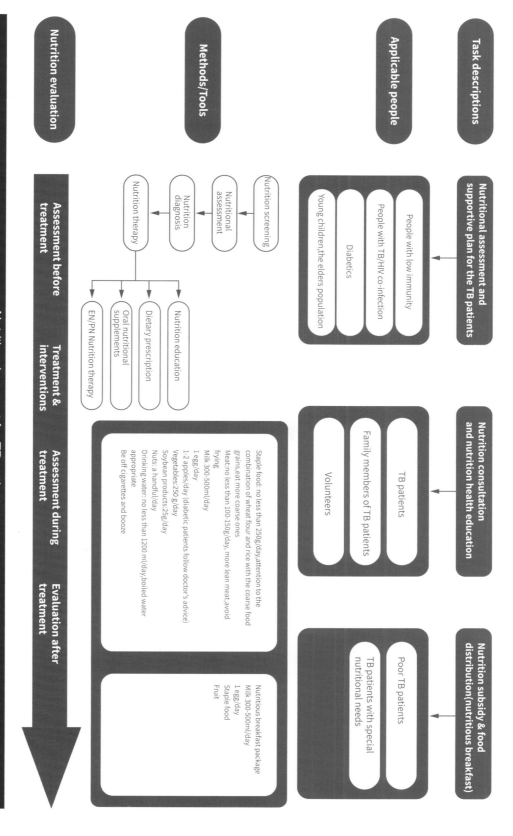

Task descriptions

| Nutritional assessment and supportive plan for the TB patients | Nutrition consultation and nutrition health education | Nutrition subsidy & food distribution(nutritious breakfast) |

Applicable people

People with low immunity
Diabetics
People with TB/HIV co-infection
Young children,the elders population

TB patients
Family members of TB patients
Volunteers

Poor TB patients
TB patients with special nutritional needs

Nutritious breakfast package
Milk 300-500ml/day
1 egg/day
Staple food
Fruit

Methods/Tools

Nutrition screening → Nutritional assessment → Nutrition diagnosis → Nutrition therapy

Nutrition therapy:
Nutrition education
Dietary prescription
Oral nutritional supplements
EN/PN Nutrition therapy

Staple food: no less than 250g/day,attention to the combination of wheat flour and rice with the coarse food grains,eat more coarse ones
Meat:no less than 100-150g/day, more lean meat,avoid frying
Milk 300-500ml/day
1 egg/day
1-2 apples/day (diabetic patients follow doctor's advice)
Vegetables-250 g/day
Soybean products:25g/day
Nuts: a handful/day
Drinking water: no less than 1200 ml/day,boiled water appropriate
Be off cigarettes and booze

Nutrition evaluation

Assessment before treatment
Treatment & interventions
Assessment during treatment
Assessment during treatment
Evaluation after treatment

Nutritional support for TB patients

45

China's tuberculosis control and prevention ecosystem

Indicators for performance check

Designated Medical institution	CDC	Comprehensive medical institution	Community medical institution
1. Etiological positive rate 2. Standard regimen utilization rate 3. Follow-up Rate 4. Treatment success rate 5. Registration management rate 6. Drug-resistance screening rate 7. Treatment rate of RR-TB patient 8. Standardized treatment rate of RR-TB patient 9. Discharge referral rate of RR-TB patient	1. Close contacts screening rate 2. Proportion of TB screening in HIV cases 3. Preventive treatment proportion in key population 4. Overall arrival rate 5. Timely response rate of pre-warning signal of single case of tuberculosis in schools 6. Coverage ratio of proficiency test for phenotypic drug sensitucity test 7. Coverage ratio of nucleic acid detection capability verification of MTB 8. Coverage ratio of rapid detection of DR genes in MTB	1. Report rate 2. Referral rate 3. Proportion of TB examination in patientswith unilateral pleural effusion 4. Proportion of TB examinationin hemoptysis patients 5. Proportion of TB screening in patients using glucocotricoids 6. Proportion of TB screening in patients using immunosuppressant 7. Culture rate 8. Proportion of patients with between initial visit to diagnosis less than 7 days	1. Regular medication rate 2. Standard management rate

Three dimensional connotation

Result	Measurement of final quality of structure and operation
Process	Quality and efficiency of dynamic operation of mechanism
Stucture	Static resource allocation relationships and efficiency

Core areas

Surveillance
- Special investigation of missing report
- Routine data check

Management
- Family doctor contract service
- Basic public health
- Whole-course management care

Diagnosis and treatment
- Outpatient standard
- Clinical pathway
- Diagnostic criteria

Laboratory
- EQA
- QA
- Biological safety

Assessment & Evaluation

Comprehensive quality control of tuberculosis control

Technical Assistant

Training